The Omni Diet Plan

High Protein Low Carb Weight Loss to Optimum Health

By Cathy Wilson
Copyright © 2013

ISBN-13:
978-1491063224

ISBN-10:
149106322X

First Printing, 2013

Printed in the United States of America

Income Disclaimer

This book contains business strategies, marketing methods and other business advice that, regardless of my own results and experience, may not produce the same results (or any results) for you. I make absolutely no guarantee, expressed or implied, that by following the advice below you will make any money or improve current profits, as there are several factors and variables that come into play regarding any given business.

Primarily, results will depend on the nature of the product or business model, the conditions of the marketplace, the experience of the individual, and situations and elements that are beyond your control.

As with any business endeavor, you assume all risk related to investment and money based on your own discretion and at your own potential expense.

Liability Disclaimer

By reading this book, you assume all risks associated with using the advice given below, with a full understanding that you, solely, are responsible for anything that may occur as a result of putting this information into action in any way, and regardless of your interpretation of the advice.

You further agree that our company cannot be held responsible in any way for the success or failure of your business as a result of the information presented in this book. It is your responsibility to conduct your own due diligence regarding the safe and successful operation of your business if you intend to apply any of our information in any way to your business operations.

Terms of Use

You are given a non-transferable, "personal use" license to this book. You cannot distribute it or share it with other individuals.

Also, there are no resale rights or private label rights granted when purchasing this book. In other words, it's for your own personal use only.

The Omni Diet Plan

High Protein Low Carb Weight Loss to Optimum Health

By Cathy Wilson

Table of Contents

Pre-Thoughts 9

How Your Body was Designed to Work 13

The Omni Diet Defined 19

The Omni Diet Historically Speaking 23

Omni Diet Basic Concepts Explained.....................27

Why go Omni? Benefits/Advantages 31

Omni "Thumbs Up" Foods 35

Omni "No-No's" 41

Sample Omni Diet Program...................................47

Diet Myths/Truths.. 51

Final Thoughts 61

Pre-Thoughts

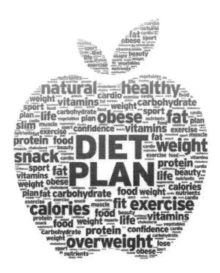

Diet is one of those words that instinctively has a negative connotation. It doesn't matter how or why you are using the word, the first thoughts are usually negative. Dieting often signifies sacrifice of some sort. Deprivation is another connective word that comes to mind.

Why is that?

It's because we are a world poisoned by a billion dollar **Fad Diet** industry. Where people are purposefully lead down a supposed magically belief that skinny, strong, and healthy, happens in a matter of days or weeks.

We all know this isn't a reality. But want so badly to believe in it that we will actually allow our mind to gather any and all false information that supports our desired believe. We can literally trick ourselves into believing that an outrageous diet plan is going to work for us, we've just got to try it one more time! The *Canadian Mental Health Association* suggests mental health is something that is important but often gets overlooked when looking to improve health.

We starve ourselves by skipping meals and not eating at all, thinking we just have to lose fat this way. This seemingly logical concept just doesn't work. What happens is your body will fight you consistently if you try. When you neglect to give your body enough of the vitamins and essential minerals it requires to function optimally, it will literally shut down on you. It doesn't trust you and why should it?

Your metabolism will lower and this means you're going to burn off fat at a lower rate than you would naturally. Not to mention the fact that every single carrot stick you ration out and give to your body is going to be stored as fat and saved for later use.

Just think of a squirrel stock piling nuts to munch on later in the winter. Your body has clicked into "starvation" mode. It will use as little energy as possible to help you function, and it's going to try and save as much energy, stored as fat, as it possibly can. Talk about mucking up your system!

By not eating your body is going to fight you and win. This will frustrate you because there will be no energy around, you're going to get sick more easily, and depression most definitely will come to light. And at the end of the tunnel there is no light because you are still going to have the same amount of fat you had before deciding to deprive your body of good health, whether you're choosing to do this through a melody of starvation tactics or just as harmful any one of ten zillion **Fad Diets**. The eating strategies just don't make sense but we try them anyway.

We've all been there and done that.

What's important is we move forward and look for ways to better ourselves; the way we eat, our lifestyle, and the way we look at life in general. Ensuring everything we do utilizes a positive perspective regardless of the circumstance. It's tough to do sometimes but definitely worth it.

Unfortunately my magic wand is in the repair shop right now and I can't get rid of the dreaded "D" word. If I could rewrite history we would call any new eating strategy a "positive lifestyle change zoning in on food." That's much, much better.

It's safe to say we can always make better food choices. The more information and knowledge we gather in this area, the better choices we can make. Taking into consideration our personal tolerances and preferences, medical history and status, genetics, lifestyle, financial status, and food knowledge to start.

I have experimented with just about every "kind" of eating out there. And yes that dates me. What I have come to realize is that we need to try it to know if we like it or not, or better yet, if we can apply a certain "type" of eating and stick with it long-term. What I'm going to help you with is to understand a fantastic route to eating well, called the Omni Diet.

It's about showing you what it's all about and most importantly how to transition your current eating style over to it and detailing why you should.

It's important you understand the basics of the Omni Diet from the ground up, so that you can be confident in your decision to stick with it. I want you to make that emotional connection because when you do there will be success.

You will look and feel fantastic. Better yet your body will be rid of the negative interferences that trigger disease and illness, and it will have all the nutrients that it requires to run effectively and efficiently for as long as it should.

This also triggers a "happy state" in your being. One that is going to be observed through your newfound level of heightened mental positivity.

You've got one life to live and the Omni Diet will help you to make the most of it.

How Your Body was Designed to Work

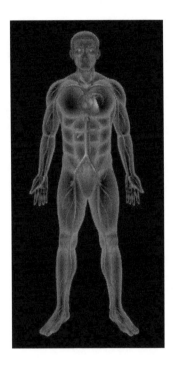

When healthy your body is an intricately designed well-oiled machine. It's made of varying systems consisting of organs that have their own specific functions. Your skin is an organ along with your heart, liver, kidneys, and bladder to start.

The five symptoms in the control center of your body are:

*Cardiovascular System
*Muscular System

*Skeletal System
*Immune System
*Endocrine System

I don't want to get in too deep here but we will touch on each of these systems just to give you a better understanding as to how your "vehicle" functions. This will help you to make the connections and manifest the reasoning as to why the Omni Diet is only going to make your systems function better.

Cardiovascular System

The circulatory system executes one main job; to ensure blood is pumped effectively throughout your body, according to *Science Daily*.

Your heart is center stage because it pumps blood through your arteries to your organs and internal systems so you can work. Your blood has hormones, oxygen, and various other nutrients that cells in your body need to grow and work properly. Your body cells use these products, at least the nutrients they require, and sends the rest out as waste in the form of carbon dioxide. Your blood will take this carbon dioxide and any other waste and rid your body of it, in theory anyway.

Muscular System

Without muscles you wouldn't be able to walk, talk, or even smile. Your skeletal muscles are attached to bones throughout your body and move by contracting and expanding. It's the smooth muscles in your digestive system that help propel water and food through it for breakdown and use. Your heart contains cardiac muscles which push oxygen and other nutrients in your blood through your body, says the experts at *Innerbody.com*.

Skeletal System

The skeletal system is configured of joints, bones, and cartilage. Cartilage has the function of helping bones and joints work more effectively united.

The functions of your bones are:

*To support your body and work with muscles to move your body, along with carrying weight.
*To protect your vital organs from being damaged. For example, your chest and rib cage help protect your lungs and heart.
*To store important vitamins and minerals like calcium and phosphorus, ready to release them when required.
*To produce blood cells.

Immune System

Your immune system helps to keep free radicals from invading and creating serious illness and disease. Bacteria, toxins, and viruses will otherwise overtake your body and take away your good health.

Your immune system is your defense to living a long and disease-free life. Your "forwards" are great eating strategies, like what you'll experience with the Omni Diet.

Lymph is a liquid made by your lymph notes that circulates through your blood and helps to keep things "clean," getting rid of harmful toxins and waste that will poison you.

In the center of your bones is bone marrow and that's where essential red and white blood cells are manufactured. Your white cells are critical because they create antibodies that look to zap toxins, bacterial, and harmful waste from your system. Think of this like you would removing negative energy. Your "thymus" is located in your chest and it manufactures special cells to help battle off disease. And your spleen works as a filter to get rid of old washed up red bloods cells and harmful entities like bacteria, according to *Healthy Living*. Your adenoids will also take part in luring in and killing harmful bacteria and viruses.

Endocrine System

The organs in this intricate system are called glands. Their function is to produce hormones, chemicals that swim through your blood and dictate to your organs what they should be doing. Body messengers are what your hormones may be called. It's your endocrine system that strives to control your mood, body development, sleep and growing rate, along with metabolism. This is the rate in which your body is able to breakdown and convert food into useable energy.

It's these five systems that dictate how your body works and these systems must receive healthy food in order to function optimally. If you feed your body "crap" all the time, it's going to work like crap. If you choose to take care of yourself by eating right, with the help of the Omni Diet, your body is going to function optimally, protecting your from disease, keeping you strong and fit, with a positive life perspective that keeps your frown turned upside down.

The Omni Diet works to give your body plenty of muscle building and energizing protein, along with all the essential vitamins and minerals it needs to keep your mind and body strong. If you listen to your body it will tell you the Omni Diet is taking you in the right direction for great health.

My Thinking . . .

Understanding how your "vehicle" works is important in the big picture of great health choices. Knowing how your body works is only going to help you connect the dots as to why your body needs certain foods and all the positive health advantages they carry. The Omni Diet focuses on delivering what you need to optimize your health; physically and mentally.

Let's look into exactly what the Omni Diet is!

The Omni Diet Defined

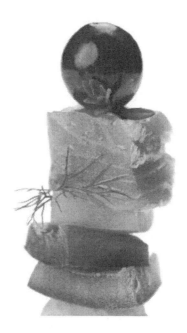

"Omnivore" defined means "eats-all or everything." Most humans eat many foods (polyphage), including numerous plants, animals fungi, and algae. Omnivores are opportunists that consume both animal protein and vegetation. Finding a balance with this eating style helps omnivores to maintain their health and wellness and remain fertile.

Understanding this helps when it comes to explaining the Omni Diet. Omni Diet is a high protein diet that stands for Optimal Macronutrient Intake Trial. Protein is an example of a macronutrient. This healthy eating strategy utilizes a high-protein diet to help level blood pressure, and is interconnected with the DASH program (Dietary Approaches to Stop Hypertension). If you can control your blood pressure naturally through food, why wouldn't you opt for this approach instead of filling your body full of harmful drugs?

Before we move further I think it's important that you understand the basics of blood pressure; what levels are safe, and the consequences of high blood pressure.

BLOOD PRESSURE LEVELS - Blood pressure readings are done by recording two numbers, systolic (top number) and diastolic (bottom number).

Systolic - Is the higher number that measures the amount of pressure in the arteries as your heart beats, or when your heart muscle is contracting.

Diastolic - This is the lower number which measures the pressure level in your arteries between each heartbeat, or as your heart muscle is taking a break and filling back up with blood.

Now we'll have a look at healthy blood pressure.

Normal - Having a systolic reading of less than 120 and a diastolic reading of less than 80.
Pre-Hypertension - Having a systolic reading of 120-139 or a diastolic reading of 80-89.
Hypertension or High Blood Pressure - *Stage One* - Your systolic is 140-159, or diastolic reading is higher than 100.
High Blood Pressure - *Stage Two* - Your systolic reading is 160 or more, and your diastolic is higher than 100.
Emergency Care Needed - If your systolic reading is more than 180 or your diastolic reading is more than 110

One reading that's abnormal doesn't mean you have high blood pressure. By having your blood pressure checked regularly you can deal with indicators of high blood pressure sooner than later.

BASIC CONSEQUENCES OF HIGH BLOOD PRESSURE

*Kidney Damage - High blood pressure will thicken and narrow blood vessels in your kidneys, forcing them to work harder regularly. The result can be they wear out and you end up with kidney failure. In basic your kidneys work to filter harmful substances from your blood.

*Stroke - People with high blood pressure have an increased risk of developing a stroke. Lowering your blood pressure is a preventable measure one can take to reduce the risk of stroke.

*Heart Disease - Uncontrolled high blood pressure is a significant factor in heart disease. It forces the heart to pump harder to get blood through your body, increasing the pressure in your arteries. Eventually the arteries will harden and get smaller, increasing pressure and preventing oxygen from getting to your heart. This means your organs will suffer and heart disease, a life-threatening condition, may develop.

The Omni Diet will help to lower your high blood pressure and this is going to help to reduce the risk of serious disease like stroke and cardiovascular disease to start.

My Thinking . . .

The Omni Diet uses a natural protein rich approach to give your body the essential nutrients it needs to function optimally. By consuming healthy fruits and vegetables your body is going to build itself strong and resistant to illness and disease. Healthy eating equates to a strong body, mind, and soul.

The Omni Diet Historically Speaking

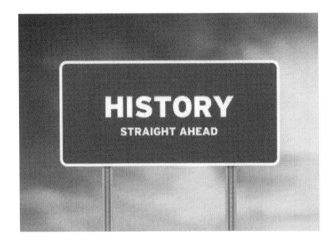

I don't think anybody is going to argue the fact that humans need food to survive, including adequate water. But from here the sky turns gray because each person seems to have different thoughts on what constitutes healthy and what doesn't, what foods are essential for good health and which aren't. And at what point is a food considered a negative rather than a positive.

In other words there has always been confusion with what specific foods your body needs in what amounts, and at what times, in order to optimize your health. Even experts that have studied nutrition for years have different "professional" opinions, which doesn't help us figure out what foods are right for us.

The Omni Heart Diet was originally created by Johns Hopkins to help manage and reduce high blood pressure. The idea was to focus on positive dietary choices to low er sodium and blood pressure. Technical this concept was referred to as the DASH or Dietary Approaches to Stop Hypertension. The team that helped Hopkins with his approach looked to study the findings of two separate clinical trials to deduce the most effective eating strategy for the plan. They concluded the best approach was a diet that lowered cholesterol and bad or saturated fat was best to help decrease blood pressure.

This is the basic history of the Omni Heart Diet anyways. That said, the Chinese have been practicing the concepts of the Omni Heart Diet for centuries and that has to account for something. Traditionally the Chinese are recognized for good health and living long and fulfilling lives. They have to be doing "something" right, and experts agree their healthy approach to eating plays a key role.

You may have also heard the Omni Diet referred to as "The Gorilla Diet." Did you know that a gorilla can eat up to forty pounds of vegetation every day? Because of this fact they really don't need to drink all that much. The vegetation they consume hydrates them naturally.

Gorillas are gigantic and strong. Their bodies are powerful and muscular. Nature's way of showing us that eating natural foods, particular plant-based, is definitely heading in the right direction for good health.

By getting back to the simple, the Omni Diet will also help you minimize or eliminate all the processed and unhealthy foods and effects from your system. That's a great place to start. And by using the Omni Diet perspective in your every day you're going to give your body what it needs to steer clear of serious disease, lower choles-

terol and high blood pressure, and help you feel ener-
gized and alive, ready to live your live to the fullest
effectively and happily.

My Thinking . . .

*The Omni Diet has been around for a while. But with so
many diet options out there, it often just gets lost in the
crowd.*

***My goal is to bring the Omni Diet to center stage so
you can decide whether or not it works for you.***

*Better yet I challenge you to find enough reasons to war-
rant not at least trying it out. History shows us what our
bodies have always needed to be healthy, resilient to
disease, and smooth and efficient in function. The Omni
Diet has a place in the history books, but's also the perfect example of food balance and better health. It's time
for you to combine simple with logic and implement the
Omni Diet.*

History says so!

Omni Diet Basic Concepts Explained

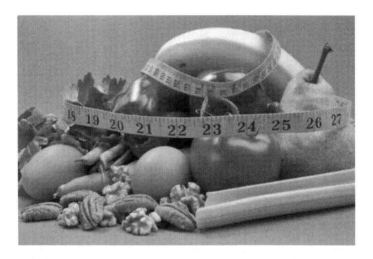

The Omni Diet is also known "slang-wise" as the Gorilla Diet and scientifically created to help people lose up to 12 pounds in just two weeks. Rather than recording all the calories you consume, which can be quite tiresome. You simply eat like a Gorilla would: lots and lots of veggies with a moderate amount of protein and a dash of nuts, seeds, and nutritious fruits.

Your body needs you to eat protein rich foods like eggs, lean meats, beans, nuts, quinoa, and tofu daily, for example, because the body doesn't manufacture or store this macronutrient. Proteins are in every cell in your body and they determine the function and health of the cell.

Other functions are:

*Cell shape and organization
*Cell manufacturing and waste cleanup

*General cell maintenance
*Regulate outside information and trigger intracellular response
*The composition of hair and nails
*Repairing and building tissue
*Manufacturing hormones, enzymes, and other body chemicals
*Building block of cartilage, muscles, bones, blood, and skin
*Gives you energy and is required to build and maintain muscle

It goes without saying your body requires large amounts of protein, a macronutrient, along with carbohydrates and fat.

Your body also needs micronutrients to stay healthy and this is where fruits and vegetables come in: loaded with essential vitamins and minerals that are necessary in small amounts. Without going into too much detail, examples of vitamins are vitamin A, B, C, D, E, and folic acid.

Some of the minerals required for great health are calcium, iron, magnesium, and zinc. Eating a diverse range of healthy foods will make sure you give your body everything it needs fuel-wise. Of course protein foods are also loaded with invaluable micronutrients for your great health.

As you already know, the Omni Diet tunes in on protein and plant balance, 30%, 70%, respectively.

Other highlights of the Omni Diet are:

*No dairy products except for organic eggs which are free range.
*Fruit juice, carbohydrates and refined sugars are eliminated.
*Soy products are removed
*Vegetable oils are eliminated, particularly those high in omega 6 fatty acid
*Processed foods should be avoided as much as possible
*High quality protein sources only
*Guidelines are to stick to the diet for at least 2 weeks so that toxins have a chance to be flushed from system
*Naturally losing fat because you are eating healthy lower-calorie foods and eliminating high-calorie, high fat processed foods
*You won't ever go hungry because food amount isn't restricted

My Thinking . . .

The Omni Diet is a simple and logical route to get your body healthy. Choosing to fuel your body with an array of tasty natural foods chalk full of essential vitamins, minerals, protein, and other nutrients is going to deter disease, clear thinking, increase your energy levels, and give you the platform in which better yourself as a whole.

Isn't that what life's all about?

Looking great, feeling great, and taking advantage of all life's opportunities at your fingertips?

The Omni Diet concept uses eating to treat and prevent illness from occurring. Everything from cancers and diabetes, to bowel issues and heart disease, this diet looks to remove the toxic triggers of sickness by eliminating the foods that aren't "right" for your body.

The tidal wave from the healthy Omni Diet is going to flush harmful toxins hiding out in our major organs, tissues and internal systems, leaving you lighter, stronger, and more optimistic in general.

The Omni Diet is just the beginning of better!

Why go Omni? Benefits/Advantages

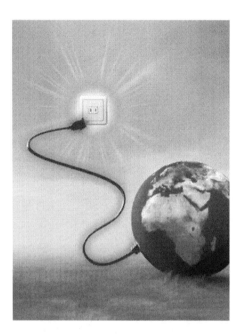

There really doesn't seem to be a "perfect" diet, one that works for every person out there. But the Omni Diet really is a fantastic choice when looking to improve your healthy for the long term.

Some of the great points of this diet are:

*It's laid out nicely and works if you stick with it
*It works nicely with the Paleo Diet, another great eating style
*The protein-plant focus is the key to naturally fast weight loss and the protein help promote fat loss not muscle loss
*Gives you plenty of energy
*Naturally helps promote weight loss

*Lowers blood pressure and cholesterol which are overt triggers of serious disease
*Helps promote better sleep, which promotes better physical and mental health
*Promotes weight loss that decreases the risk of serious disease, improves mood, decreases aches and pain, and boosts self-confidence
*Natural decrease is inflammation
*Sharper brain function
*Quality calories that fill you up
*Wide diversity of nutrients
*Decreased feelings of hunger
*Leveling of hormones, improving the odds of breaking unhealthy food addictions
*Increased feeling of wellness
*Plant-based foods fight off illness/disease

The Omni Diet produces the perfect balance of fruits, nuts, vegetables, fish, and lean meats to give your body exactly what it needs to lose weight, build healthy and strong lean muscle, and to promote long-term growth and well-being.

My Thinking . . .

The advantages of the Omni Diet are deep and wide. It will help to build your mind and body strong, which is only going to help you prepare to tackle life challenges head on. Your body was built to thrive with "natural" food choices. It has always needed plenty of vegetables, healthy lean meats, and all the essential vitamins and minerals that come with natural eating, according to experts at Livestrong.

Unfortunately somewhere along the road of life we let external stimuli interfere with good eating, and the result just isn't pretty. Obesity, stroke, diabetes, cardiovascular disease, and various mental illnesses are directly linked to poor eating habits accumulated over time. The Omni Diet is your tool to break these bad eating habits and slowly but surely get your great health back.

The choice is yours.

You can continue to life as you are and sell yourself short. Or you can think long and hard about the positive advantages of the Omni Diet and commit to making the "right" choice. It's the one that only leads to bigger in better in everything.

Omni "Thumbs Up" Foods

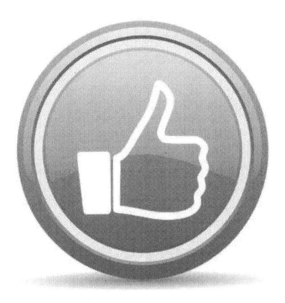

As you already know the Omni Diet focuses on **LOTS** of vegetables and a good amount of protein. The theory is these food categories will give your body all the nutrients it requires to build itself strong and resilient to disease.

We all have to eat to live and unfortunately with life so technically stressed and food so readily available, many of us get unhealthy and create the reality of living to eat.

We stop listening to our body and allow external factors, boredom, stress, and social pressures to interfere with our once healthy eating. We often interconnect eating with emotion and more often than not we get caught on the roller coaster of unhealthy eating and overall poor health. Comfort foods end up establishing themselves into our everyday eating habits. Simple carb options like sweet pastries, chips, chocolate bars and cakes become our emotional outlets. It's a quick sugar high that quickly drops us into the depths of despair when our blood sugar levels plummet. High fat trans-fat food options take center stage in our lives for convenience, economic reasons, created comfort, and their addictive nature. Sort of like the "forbidden fruit" if you will. And it doesn't take long for poor food choices to transform into habit.

The Omni Diet teaches us that healthy eating doesn't mean sacrifice or not looking forward to eating. It's about common sense eating. Fueling your body with "smart" choices that are going to help you live longer, look great, and feel fabulous.

Here are the foods that the Omni Diet knows are going to help you get healthy and happy fast and for the long-run.

MEATS (4 oz. / serving) (broiled, grilled, barbecued, steamed or baked)
-beef
-veal
-buffalo
-chicken (skinless)
-flounder
-Chilean sea bass
-halibut
-sole
-shrimp
-lobster

VEGETABLES (1 cup / serving) (raw, steam, grilled or boiled)
-broccoli

-fresh green beans
-chard
-spinach
-beets
-lettuce
-tomatoes
-celery
-carrots
-onion
-jalapenos
-fennel
-asparagus
-cucumber
-radishes
-cabbage
-peppers
-peas
-Brussels sprouts
-celery
-eggplant

DRESSING
-apple cider vinegar
-seasoned lemon

FRUIT
-orange
-apple
-grapefruit
-strawberries
-blueberries
-blackberries
-banana
-peach
-plum
-nectarine
-pineapple

-cantaloupe
-watermelon
-musk melon
-pear
-apricot
-grapes
-star fruit
-tangerine

NUTS/SEEDS
-peanuts
-sunflower seeds
-flaxseed
-poppy seeds
-sesame seeds
-walnuts
-almonds
-macadamia nuts
-fennel
-pecans
-pine nuts
-pistachio
-pumpkin seeds
-quinoa
-cashews
-hazelnuts
-corn nuts
-mustard seed

DRINKING
-water
-black coffee
-herbal tea
-lemon water
-vegetable juice

My Thinking . . .

The idea is to eat tons of vegetables and veggie juice each day, healthy amounts of lean meats, and minimal amounts of nuts, seeds, and fruits. This will guide your body back to a normal and energizing state of wellness.

Omni "No-No's"

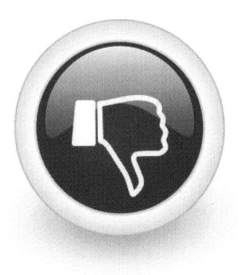

The majority of foods bought at the grocery store, from cheese and cookies, to crackers and lunch snacks, are called processed food.

WebMD experts state processed foods are directly linked to obesity, heart disease, stroke, diabetes, and other serious preventable diseases.

Processed or fabricated food is not natural when you buy it. You won't find these foods naturally available on earth, like you would oranges or squash.

In the eyes of the Omni Diet these foods that aren't natural should be avoided, because the body isn't designed to break these foods down.

The foods to avoid are:

-dairy
-processed packaged and fast foods
-sugars
-grains

WHY NO DAIRY?

Naturally an elephant will nurse her young calf as their main source of nutrition. The same goes for a baby boy or girl. It's scientifically proven breast milk is the optimum source of nutrition for at least the first six months. You don't see heifers or cows drinking milk, or any other mammals, except maybe atypical cats, dogs, and rabbits on a farm, and that's a whole other book!

Dairy Truths

*Milk does not reduce the chance of fracturing a bone.
*Less milk or dairy means less bone breaks.
*It's the Vitamin D and not the calcium that deters fractures.
*Calcium may raise the risk of prostate cancer.
*Calcium does benefits colon cancer.
*Up to 75% of the world population is lactose intolerant and can't process dairy, according to *Prevention Magazine*.

Dairy Might Also Be Linked To:

*Sinus Issues
*Allergies
*Type 1 Diabetes
*Anemia
*Constipation

42

*Ear Infections

WHY NO PROCESSED FOODS?

Processed foods are anything but simple. Many are loaded with addictive trans-fat or "fake" fat because it makes food taste good, increases shelf life, and is cheap for the manufacturer.

A few other reasons processed foods aren't the best choice are:

*They have fewer nutrients and more additives
*Lots of harmful "fat" is added
*Sugars and sugar substitute is also added
*They have synthetic vitamins and minerals added

Anything that comes in a "package" per say, is considered a processed food. Processed foods are linked to obesity and pretty much every condition, illness, and disease under the sun, and all of this has been scientifically proven.

WHY NO SUGARS?

Sugar gives your body the glucose it requires for energy. There are natural sugars in fruit for example, makes it sweet and yummy. That's healthy for you in small doses. The trouble arises when sugar is added to foods. This has a negative effect on your health. Just think cakes, pastries, cookies, pies, and chocolate bars.

I don't want to get too detailed here so we'll just talk about the two main kinds of carbohydrates for an example; complex and simple.

Complex Carbohydrates have lots of fiber and nutrients, along with some sugar, and they take longer to break down, giving your system energy that lasts. Complex carbohydrates are found in foods like whole grain breads and cereals, whole wheat pasta and rice, and sweet potatoes.

Foods like cakes, muffins, soda, cookies, chocolate bars, chips and other packaged sweets, along with white bread, pasta and rice, are simple sugars. They cause the blood sugar levels to spike in your system because they are short term energy. This triggers your mood to fluctuate and energy levels will go from sky high one minute straight to the bottom of the barrel next.

I don't want to confuse you but natural vegetables, fruits, nuts, whole grains, and beans all contain simple sugars.

But these "natural" simple sugars also come with protein, fiber, vitamins, minerals and phytochemicals, all things your body requires for optimum function. So it's the unnatural foods with simple sugars that you want to avoid.

They are only going to wreak havoc with your mind and body, interfering with your natural systems, triggering sleep issues, mental stress, obesity, self-confidence issues, and serious disease to start.

Specialty Note: Simple sugars that are unnatural are consumed in excess have been shown to trigger serious preventable disease like type 2 diabetes.

Experts believe the constant spikes in blood sugars trigger this disease and encourage its development.

The Omni Diet steers clear of these harmful sugars and has been known to prevent, better, and even reverse type 2 diabetes.

WHY NO GRAINS?

By cutting these foods out you will reduce inflammation, and better or even reverse disease like diabetes, obesity, chronic pain, chronic fatigue syndrome, immune disorders, bowel disease, and so many more.

My Thinking . . .

By removing the foods from your system that are causing interference with your good health, you're making room for all the essential nutrients to be utilized.

The body wasn't designed to process the "fake" processed foods humans created. And there are some "natural" foods, like milk, that is designed for the first phase in life as a newborn, but not necessary later in life.

The Omni diet uses common sense and scientific evidence to ensure you get everything your body needs and not the foods that are harmful as a whole.

Are you going to put gasoline in your diesel tractor? *I did by mistake as a kid but you're not.*

So why would you put harmful food into your belly?

Just something to ponder…

Sample Omni Diet Program

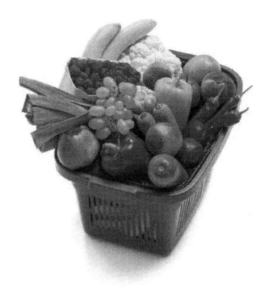

The Omni Diet program is a 6 week starter divided into four phases. This will get you set up to stick with the Omni for life! We'll have a look at sample food items you should have on your shopping list and a sample day of meal planning just to give you an idea.

SHOPPING LIST

Meats - You want to choose healthy organic, free-range, with no hormones or antibiotics, and "wild" is good.

*chicken and turkey (skinless)
*tuna and wild salmon
*bison
*herring

*shrimp and mackerel
*lamb

Veggies - Here you want organic and fresh as much as you can.

*Brussels sprouts
*broccoli
*chard
*Bok Choy
*sweet Potato
*green Beans
*peas
*carrots
*celery

*eggplant
*mushrooms
*onions
*cabbage
*tomatoes
*peppers
*spinach
*avocado
*zucchini

Fridge and Cupboard Starters

*salsa, hummus, guacamole
*eggs, organic, free-range
*herbs and spices
*almond butter and coconut butter
*meat (lean)
*coconut oil, olive oil
*almond milk, coconut milk
*good protein powder
*coconut wraps
*seeds and nuts
*quinoa
*fresh and frozen organic fruits, berries in particular
*pomegranate, macra root and lacuna (super foods)
*fresh organic produce - no white potato
*stevia and erythritol for sweetening
*vegannaise

Spices - fresh and organic is best

*pepper
*oregano
*basil
*mint
*ginger
*cinnamon
*garlic
*cumin
*dill
*thyme

SAMPLE DAY

Meal 1 Breakfast

1 egg poached (2 for guys)
2 cups cooked spinach
1/2cup fresh berries

Snack

1 tomato sliced
1/4 cup avocado
Raw veggies

Meal 2 Lunch

1 grilled chicken breast
2 cups Romaine lettuce
Tomatoes, cucumber, alfalfa sprouts, carrots, peppers
Seasoned lemon juice

Snack

1/4 cup mixed nuts/seeds
1 piece fresh fruit

Meal 3 Dinner

Barbecued salmon steak
Grilled sweet potato
Steamed mixed veggies (broccoli, Bok Choy, celery, onion, eggplant, zucchini, tomato), and sunflower seeds

My Thinking . . .

Keep in mind this is just to get you started. You will discover with time your preferences and tolerances, and most definitely expand on your shopping list and the meals in which you come to love.

The Omni Diet really isn't that difficult if you think about it. The shopping list makes sense. If you pick up a food item at the grocery store that is in a package with ingredients you can't pronounce, put it back. You need to stick with natural foods.

Front and center are fresh vegetables, followed by wholesome, organic lean meats, and nuts, seeds, and fruits.

***BONUS** - You'll never go hungry because your body always needs constant refueling with nutritious and natural food choices.*

Don't you think it's time for you to start listening to your body and delivering?

Diet Myths/Truths

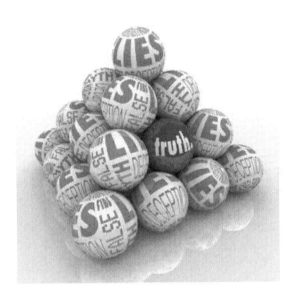

MYTH 1 - Low-fat diets are the best route to lose weight fast and get healthy.

TRUTH - Unfortunately our fabricated society supports this notion but it really couldn't be further from the truth. We shouldn't be afraid of fat because without it we wouldn't be alive, according to experts at *Science Daily*. Your body needs up to 30% of its calories from fat, and uses it to give you energy and metabolize certain vitamins and minerals effectively.

However, it's the **type** of fat you ingest that's critical. Most saturated fats found in ice cream, butter, and cheese, are not healthy for your system. Along with dangerous Trans fats that are hidden in processed foods like packaged cakes, muffins, cookies, and crackers. These

51

fats your body can't process properly and they end up triggering all sorts of health issues, starting with obesity.

Unsaturated fats in moderation are what your body needs, like the fat in olive oil, sunflower oil, or avocado, says the nutritionists at *T*.

MYTH 2 - Starving yourself will help you lose weight fast.

TRUTH - If you are trying to lose weight fast by starving yourself skipping meals, or not eating enough food, this won't help you. In fact it'll hinder your weight loss efforts.

If you starve yourself your body will literally start to shut down and take every single carrot stick you eat and store it as fat. You've put your body into defense mode. It doesn't trust you and is trying to store fat so you can survive the times you decide to neglect your body the nutrients it requires to perform optimally.

Not eating lowers your metabolism, the rate in which you burn calories, which slows or stops fat loss. You are also going to force your body to burn muscle for energy instead of fat simply because if you aren't eating regularly your body isn't getting enough protein to give you energy and keep your body strong.

VIP - Protein isn't made by your body nor can your body store it. This means if you aren't eating enough you are forcing your body to break down the muscle you already worked hard to build in order to function. If you neglect your body it will choose to burn muscle over fat. Talk about a double whammy!

You need to eat to lose weight!

It's not necessarily how much you eat but what food choices you make. By choosing to eat healthy and balanced meals, like the Omni Diet, you're going to give your body the macronutrients and micronutrients it requires to keep your body and mind strong, fit, and burn off that excess fat for life, not just a few months.

MYTH 3 - If you have a slower metabolism you are never going to lose fat.

TRUTH - Every person is different. The rate in which you burn calories is dependent on various factors, including:

*genetics
*body composition
*lifestyle
*exercise habits
*overall health
*nutrition

If you are larger you'll naturally burn more calories than a smaller person. This doesn't mean the smaller person can't lose fat. By eating natural and nutritious foods in the right amounts and exercising regularly, fat just isn't going to stand a chance regardless.

MYTH 4 - If you're going to have sweets it should be before a meal when you're truly hungry.

TRUTH - You certainly weren't born craving sweet! At some point in life you created the habit and just went with it. Having sweets when your tummy is rumbling teaches your body to crave sweet every single time you are hungry, which of course is not a good thing. This doesn't mean you can't ever have a sweet.

If you truly want a sweet you should wait until you've filled your belly full of healthy food choices. If the **want** is still there, you can have a little treat without making it habit.

MYTH 5 - If you eat later at night you are going to store more fat.

TRUTH - You might believe this but it's just not true. Studies show it's **what** you eat and **how much** you eat that determines if you are going to gain fat or not. Typically people opt for the junk food at night that contributes directly to obesity if it becomes habit.

So it makes sense you would **think** late night eating means more fat. For optimum health you're best to spread your nutritious foods out evenly throughout the day because this is when you usually exert most of your energy, according to *Men's Fitness*. Steer clear of late night junk food snacking and keep fat away.

MYTH 6 - When you stop smoking you get fat.

TRUTH - It's true that smoking does increase your metabolism slightly and this means you are burning more calories. But the amount is so minimal that quitting doesn't make you fat.

What makes you fat is making unhealthy food choices and not exercising regularly. The Omni diet helps you filter those harmful carcinogens out of your organs and internal systems by overloading you with essential vitamins, minerals, and nutrients your body needs to get healthy

MYTH 7 - Caffeine is unhealthy.

TRUTH - Fact is there are studies that show caffeine could have a positive benefit with regards to certain disease, like Parkinson's and gout. Keep in mind moderation here though because there's such thing as too much of a good thing.

Note - Caffeine does **NOT** dehydrate you as many people think. 1-2 glasses a day might very well be beneficial to your overall good health.

MYTH 8 - It's imperative to take vitamin and mineral supplements if you want to be healthy.

TRUTH - Vitamin and mineral supplements can't replace the real thing, which of course is getting these essential nutrients from all the "right" foods. Fiber, complex carbohydrates, lean protein, essential fats, and numerous other nutrients need to come from healthy and well-balanced food choices for the most part.

EXCEPTION - You may have some health issues that deter your body from absorbing a particular nutrient, which means supplementation may be your only option.

Bottom line is to do whatever it takes to give your body the nutrition it requires. Just make sure Plan A is **real** food and Plan B supplements is a backup.

MYTH 9 - Energy drinks are the fastest route to get your body up and running.

TRUTH - Energy drinks are **NOT** the route to go if you're dragging your butt. Sure you might feel like you're on cloud ten for a short while after, but the crash that's coming just isn't fun.

Did you know that **ONE** energy drink can have up to 14 teaspoons of sugar, according to *Diabetes Association of Canada*?

Yikes! Add to that a large dose of caffeine and you're walking on thin ice...**DANGER!**

MYTH 10 - Consuming too much sugar will lead to diabetes.

FACT - You aren't going to get diabetes from having too much sugar. However, if you continuously make un-healthy food choices that are loaded with sugar, ones that are low in nutritional content and high in calories, you will inevitably gain weight and this will increase your risk of developing preventable diabetes.

Other factors to take into consideration are:

*current health
*genetics
*family history
*lifestyle
*nutrition
*exercise habits

MYTH 11 - To limit your sodium intake, then just stop using the salt shaker.

TRUTH - Pointing the finger is easy. In large part the ex-cess sodium we consume is from processed foods, eating out, and packaged foods. In fact up to 75% of "ex-tra" salt comes from these sources, according to experts at *Canadian Living*.

By limiting or eliminating processed foods and opting for "au natural," instead of restaurant and packaged fuel, you

WILL lower your overall sodium and better your overall health in one foul swoop. The Omni diet is a fantastic route to purge your body of too much salt and helping you to find your balance.

MYTH 12 - Fruit isn't healthy for you because it has too much sugar.

TRUTH - Sure fruit naturally has lots of sweet sugars, but it's a healthy food choice. Fruit is loaded with essential vitamins and minerals and antioxidants that help protect from disease by zapping harmful free-radicals in their tracks.

Vegetables are a better choice than fruit, but the latter is a close second. It's much better to have a piece of fresh fruit or bowl of mixed berries than a chocolate bar, candy, or a soft drink. Two or three servings a day of fresh fruit is all good in the big book of great health. The Omni Diet supports this truth, a truth that makes perfect sense.

MYTH 13 - You should limit your tea drinking because it will dehydrate you.

TRUTH - Often tea is interlinked with coffee myths. Which makes people falsely believe tea is dehydrating.

Herbal teas are your best choice because they don't contain any caffeine and are pretty much level with water, the best option for drinking. Some teas have caffeine in them but it is so minimal this doesn't merit any worrying.

Whether hot or cold tea is another great option for wetting your whistle and keeping your body hydrated and ready to tackle any obstacle in your way.

MYTH 14 - You don't have to worry about your sodium intake unless you have high blood pressure.

TRUTH - Bottom line is as a society we get way too much salt. It makes perfect sense that everyone can benefit for reducing the amount of sodium they get. Eating too much sodium can cause all sorts of trouble with your healthy, including:

*high blood pressure
*kidney disease
*stroke
*cardiovascular disease

In general we need about 1500 mg/day of sodium, according to *Pediatricians of America*. Experts say most of us get at least double that. The Omni Diet doesn't focus on sodium intake but rather eating healthy as a whole. By consuming natural foods to fuel your body you're going to naturally lower your sodium intake drastically. This is only going to better your health.

MYTH 15 - You MUST drink 8 glasses of water every day to be hydrated.

TRUTH - There is no scientific truth to prove this. Of course water is vital to your good health and it is the best choice for quenching your thirst.

There are other liquids that can also do the trick nicely; like herbal tea and clear soups.

How much water you need is different from person to person. If you are larger and incredibly active you're going to need more liquid than someone that is smaller and less active. The environment also comes into play here. If you live in a hot place you're naturally going to need more water than someone that lives in a colder environment. The key here is to take your personal circumstance into consideration. If it suddenly gets smoking hot out, make sure you increase your liquid intake. The same goes for if you start a new exercise routine that gets your body sweating. Be smart and hydrate yourself.

My Thoughts . . .

There are so many rumors floating around with regards to health and wellness. It's important to have accurate information when you are figuring out the best lifestyle changes for you.

If you don't base your food decision on fact, how can you expect to make the "right" ones? Well you just can't.

Hopefully now you have a little more clarity on what's true and what isn't when it comes to eating and your great health. The Omni Diet really does make sense.

It uses common sense, scientific evidence, and a natural and simple approach to get your health and wellness on track for life. It's not a "one-hit-wonder" that always comes back around.

The Omni Diet is a launch pad that's only going to improve your life as a whole. That's a fact.

Health Alert: Omni Diet Sees Big Picture

Better mind, better body, better attitude, and better life are what the Omni Diet is all about. This simple plan offers disease-fighting foods from natural fuel sources, along with lean protein to keep your muscles strong and thinking sharp.

The perfect balance for optimum results is 70% plant protein and 30% lean protein. With the ultimate goals of:

*Restoring energy balance
*Decreasing the risk of disease
*Reversing some illnesses/disease
*Promoting weight loss
*Improving self-confidence

The Omni Diet isn't a quick fix fad diet. Rather a positive life change that's going to build your body strong from the inside-out.

Final Thoughts

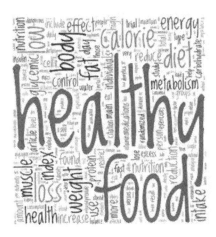

I can honestly say that out of all the diets I have studied, experienced and reflected on, the Omni Diet ranks tops in just making sense. Sure there's always a learning curve to start. But with a base knowledge and the direction to apply, the Omni Diet really is the easiest and most beneficial route for you to reach your optimum health level, regardless of your knowledge base or life situation.

The Omni Diet has everything your body needs and craves to zap dangerous free-radicals, fill you full of energy, help you lose excess fat, and finally find the eating style that you are going to want to stick with for life.

This isn't a trial "diet," it's so much more than that.

If you are serious about great health, and if you value your life and appreciate all the opportunities it has to offer ,then you'd truly be nuts to ignore the Omni way of eating. Commit to it for just 6 weeks.

If you do this I can pretty much guarantee you'll be kicking yourself in the butt for not trying it sooner.

Maybe the best time to test the waters of the Omni Diet was ten or twenty years ago, so what?

The next best time is right now. No excuses. I've given you the basics you need to decide whether the Omni Diet is "right" for you.

I'll stop yammering now so you can get started!

Thanks for reading!

And finally...

We have the choice to look for the positive or the negative in life. You can choose to lift someone up or to stomp on them. Writing is my passion and I work hard at it. With the goal of helping make people better.

If you gain a new piece of knowledge, read something that makes you think, or perhaps even smile a few times, then I am one happy camper!

Life's just too short not to tune into optimism. If your glass is half full then I invite you to read my writing. And if you have a minute to spare when you're through, **I would appreciate your review.**

This will help me better myself and my writing.

I thank you in advance and appreciate you.

Last Thoughts…

*THANK-YOU for reading my masterpiece. I hope you learned a little something, or at least got a few smiles.
*I would appreciate a millisecond or three of your time for a quick review, to help me build my masterful book empire higher.
*Whatever you do, don't forget to smile, and of course, check out my website for more of my e-Book masterpieces!
http://www.flawlesscreativewriting.com

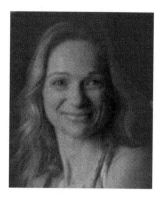

Cathy☺

Printed in Great Britain
by Amazon